The Smart Keto Vegetarian Cookbook

Easy, Mouthwatering and Affordable Keto Vegetarian Recipes to Lose Weight and Feel Great

Lidia Wong

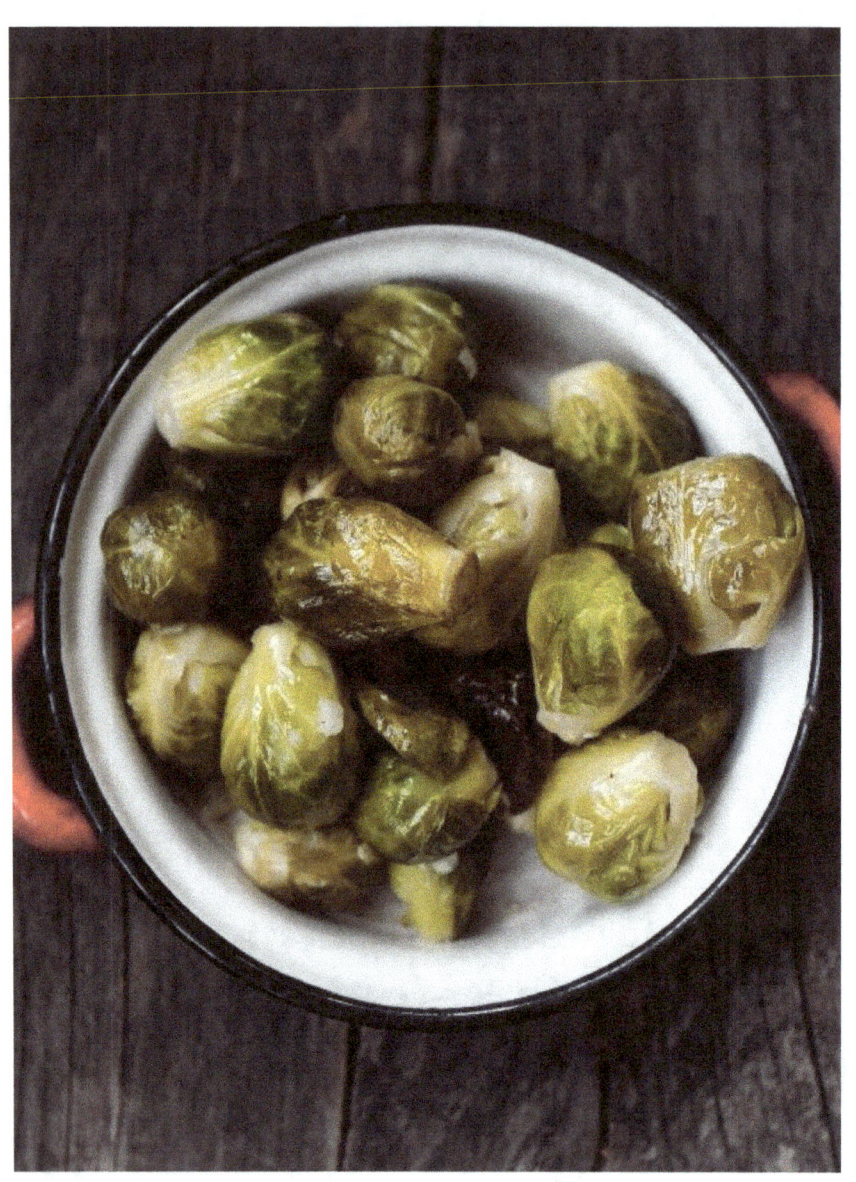

© **Copyright 2021 by Lidia Wong - All rights reserved.**

The content contained within this book may not be reproduced, duplicated or transmitted without direct written permission from the author or the publisher.

Under no circumstances will any blame or legal responsibility be held against the publisher, or author, for any damages, reparation, or monetary loss due to the information contained within this book. Either directly or indirectly.

Legal Notice:

This book is copyright protected. This book is only for personal use. You cannot amend, distribute, sell, use, quote or paraphrase any part, or the content within this book, without the consent of the author or publisher.

Disclaimer Notice:

Please note the information contained within this document is for educational and entertainment purposes only. All effort has been executed to present accurate, up to date, and reliable, complete information. No warranties of any kind are declared or implied. Readers acknowledge that the author is not engaging in the rendering of legal, financial, medical or professional advice. The content within this book has been derived from various sources. Please consult a licensed professional before attempting any techniques outlined in this book.

By reading this document, the reader agrees that under no circumstances is the author responsible for any losses, direct or indirect, which are incurred as a result of the use of information contained within this document, including, but not limited to, — errors, omissions, or inaccuracies.

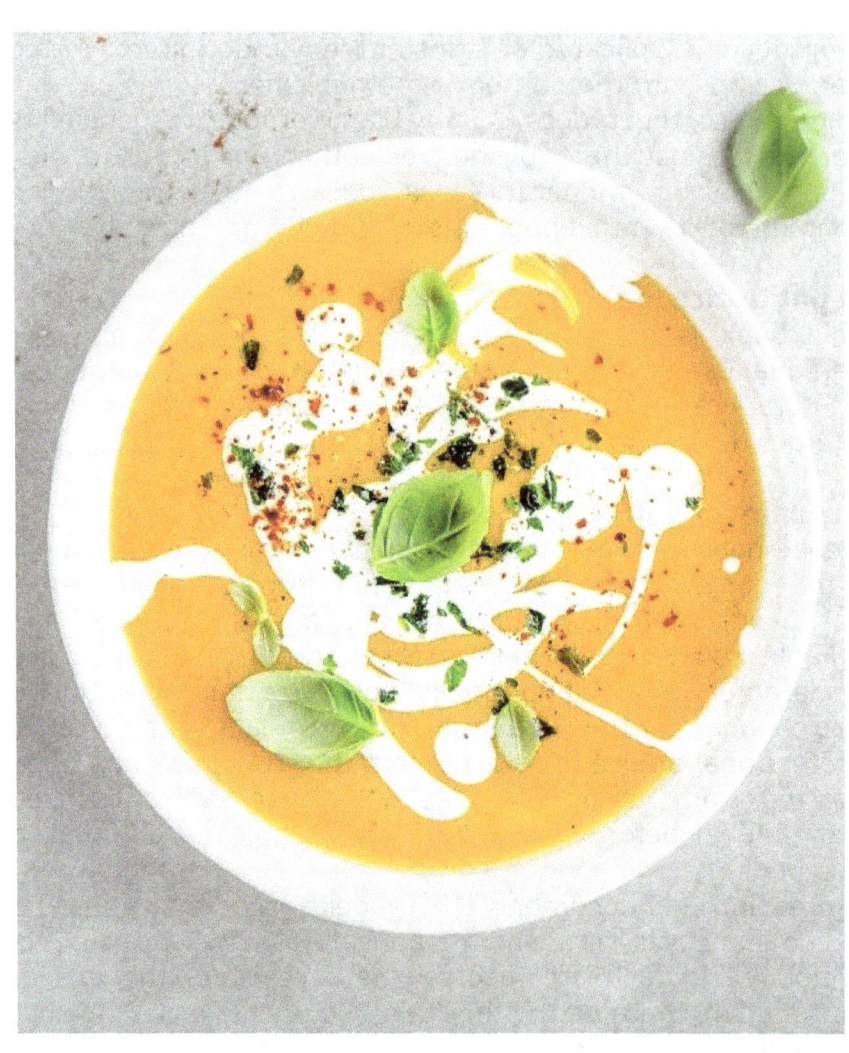

TABLE OF CONTENTS

INTRODUCTION 1

Creamy Zucchini Noodles 3

Vegetarian Keto Breakfast Frittata 6

Kale and Cucumber Salad 8

Collard Greens and Garlic Mix 9

Cauliflower Rice and Chia Mix 10

Creamy Onion Soup 12

Creamy Cucumber Egg Salad 14

Coconut Broccoli Cheese Loaf 15

Creamy Egg Salad 16

Avocado Coconut Pie 18

Mushroom Rice 21

Sage Quinoa 23

Mushroom And Peas Risotto 24

Brussels Sprouts 26

Italian Veggie Side Dish 28

Roasted Artichokes and Sauce 30

Sage Pecan Cauliflower 32

Ratatouille (Pressure cooker) 34

Creamy Garlic-Spinach Rotini Soup 36

Italian Wedding Soup 38

Tomato Orzo Soup 40

Golden Potato Soup 42

Coconut and Curry Soup 44

Spicy Black Bean Orzo Soup 46

Minestrone 48

Black And Gold Gazpacho 51

Parsley-Lime Pasta 53

Creamy Seitan Shirataki Fettucine 55

Tomato Avocado Cucumber Salad 58

Avocado Almond Cabbage Salad 60

Rich Chickpeas And Lentils Soup 62

Not-Tuna Salad 64

Red Bean and Corn Salad 66

Roasted Beet and Avocado Salad 68

Deconstructed Hummus Pitas 70

Mushroom Cakes 72

Arugula Dip 74

Basil Eggplant Tapenade 75

Green Beans Dip 77

Brussels sprouts Chips 79

Quinoa and Black Bean Burgers 81

Chocolate And Walnut Farfalle 83

Almond-Date Energy Bites 84

Melon Coconut Mousse 86

Chia Seeds Pudding with Berries 87

Dates and Cocoa Bowls 89

Blackberries Brownies 90

Rhubarb Stew 92

Cocoa Cream 94

Cloud Bread 96

Simple Almond Butter Fudge 98

Choco Chia Pudding 99

NOTE **101**

INTRODUCTION

The keto diet is the shortened term for ketogenic diet and it is essentially a high-fat and low-carb diet that helps you lose weight, thereby bringing various health benefits. This diet drastically restricts your carb intake while increasing your fat intake; this pushes your body to go into a state know as "*ketosis*". We will tackle ketosis in a bit.

The human body uses glucose from carbs to fuel metabolic pathways—meaning various bodily functions like digestion, breathing, etc.. Essentially, anything that needs energy. Even when you are resting, the body needs fuel or energy for you to continue living. If you think about it, when have you ever stopped breathing, or your heart stopped beating, or your liver stopped from cleansing the body, or your kidneys from filtering blood?

Never, unless you're dead, which is the only time in which the body doesn't need energy. In normal circumstances, glucose is the primary pathway when it comes to sourcing the body's energy.

But the body also has another pathway; it can utilize fats to fuel the various bodily processes. And this is what we call "*ketosis*". And the body can only enter ketosis when there is no glucose available, thus the reason for sticking to a low-carb diet is essential in the keto diet. Since no glucose is available, the body is pushed to use fats—it can either come from the food you consume or from your body's fat reserves—the adipose tissue or from the flabby parts of your body. This is how the keto diet helps you lose weight, by burning up all those stored fats that you have and using it to fuel bodily processes.

That said, if for whatever reason you are a vegetarian, following a ketogenic diet can be extremely difficult. A vegetarian diet is largely free of animal products, which means that food tends to be usually high in carbohydrates. Still, with careful planning, it is possible. This Cookbook will provide you with various easy and delicious dishes to help you stick to your ketogenic diet plan while being a vegetarian.

Enjoy!

Creamy Zucchini Noodles

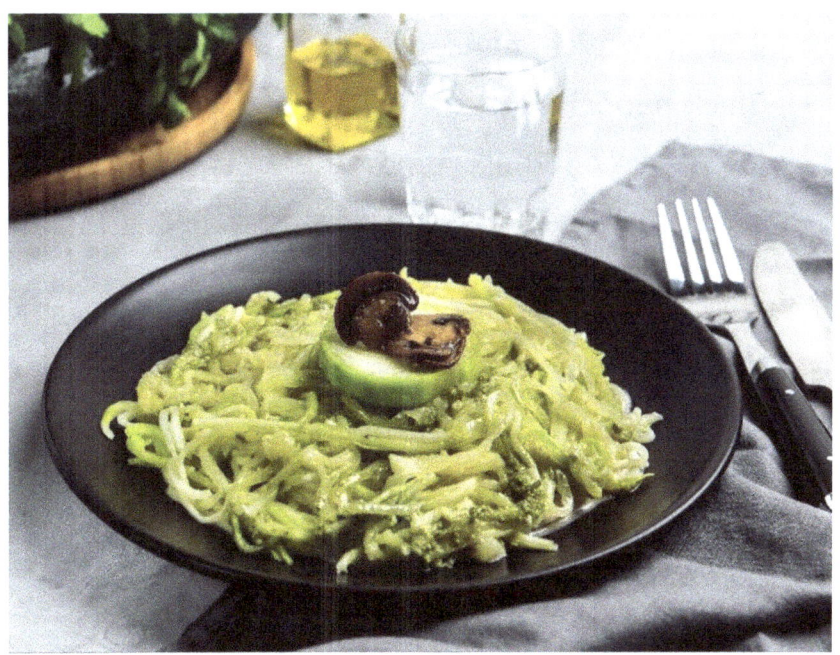

Preparation Time: 10 minutes

Cooking Time: 5 minutes

Servings: 4

Ingredients:

- 3 medium zucchinis, use spiralizer to make noodles

- 1 tablespoon arrowroot powder
- ¼ teaspoon ground nutmeg
- 1 teaspoon butter
- 2 garlic cloves, minced
- Black pepper to taste
- ½ cup almond milk, unsweetened
- ¾ cup parmesan cheese, grated

Directions:

1. In a pan over medium-high heat melt butter.
2. Add in the garlic and cook for about 1 minute or until garlic softens.
3. Decrease the heat to medium-low.
4. Add heavy cream, almond milk, nutmeg and stir well, bringing to a simmer.
5. In a mixing bowl, whisk 2 tablespoons of water and arrowroot powder until smooth.
6. Pour mixture into the pan and stir well.
7. Add black pepper and grated cheese and stir until cheese melts.
8. Pour sauce into a bowl, cover and set aside.
9. Heat pan over medium-high heat.

10. Once the pan is hot adding in zucchini noodles and stir until they soften, for about 5 minutes.
11. Now stir in the prepared sauce and serve.

Nutritional Values (Per Serving):

Calories: 307 Fat: 21.9 g Carbohydrates: 9.2 g Sugar: 3.6 g Protein: 20.6 g Cholesterol: 33 mg

Vegetarian Keto Breakfast Frittata

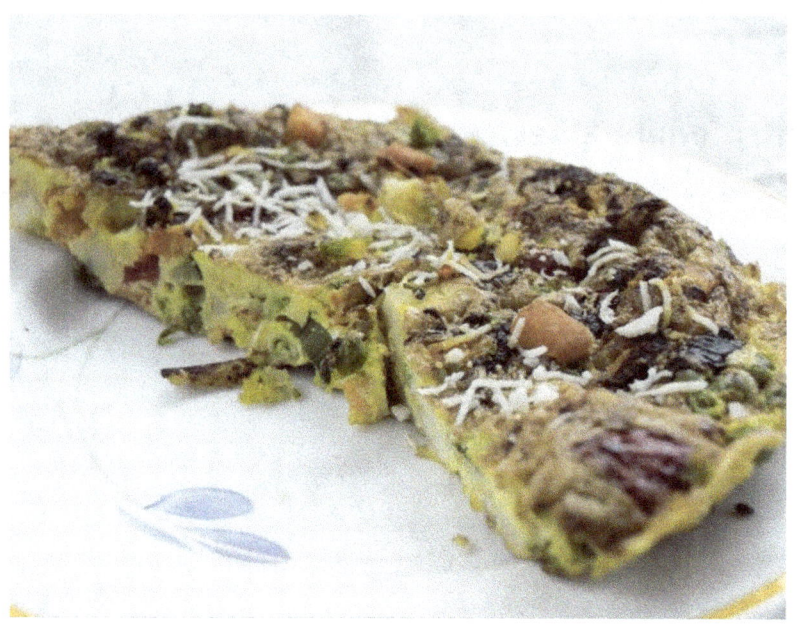

Preparation Time: 10 minutes

Cooking Time: 5 minutes

Servings: 4

Ingredients:

- 4 organic eggs
- ¼ teaspoon sea salt
- 2-ounces cheddar cheese, shredded

- 1 avocado, peeled, sliced
- 10 olives, pitted
- 1 teaspoon herb de Provence
- 2 tablespoons olive oil
- 2 tablespoons butter

Directions:

1. In a mixing bowl, add herb de Provence, eggs, olives, sea salt and whisk until frothy. Melt the butter in a pan over high heat.
2. Add avocado slices to pan and cook until lightly golden brown. Remove from pan and set aside.
3. Pour the egg mixture into the pan and sprinkle cheese on top over the top of egg mixture.
4. Cover pan with lid and cook for 3 minutes. Flip over to other side and cook for another 2 minutes.
5. Transfer the frittata to serving plate and top with avocado slices. Enjoy!

Nutritional Values (Per Serving):

Calories: 346 Fat: 32.8 g Carbohydrates: 5.5 g Sugar: 0.7 g Protein: 10.2 g Cholesterol: 194 mg

Kale and Cucumber Salad

Preparation time: 10 minutes

Cooking time: 0 minutes

Servings: 4

Ingredients:

- 2 cucumbers, sliced
- 2 cups baby kale
- 2 tablespoons avocado oil
- 1 teaspoon balsamic vinegar
- 1 cup coconut cream
- 2 tablespoons dill, chopped

Directions:

1. In a bowl, combine the kale with the cucumbers and the other ingredients, toss and serve.

Nutrition:

Calories 90, fat 1, fiber 3, carbs 7, protein 2

Collard Greens and Garlic Mix

Preparation time: 10 minutes

Cooking time: 10 minutes

Servings: 4

Ingredients:

- 2 tablespoons avocado oil
- 1 tomato, cubed
- 4 garlic cloves, minced
- 4 bunches collard greens
- A pinch of sea salt and black pepper
- Black pepper to the taste
- 1 tablespoon almonds, chopped

Directions:

1. Heat up a pan with the oil over medium heat, add the garlic, collard greens and the other ingredients, toss well, cook for 10 minutes, divide into bowls and serve.

Nutrition:

Calories 130, fat 1, fiber 8, carbs 10, protein 6

Cauliflower Rice and Chia Mix

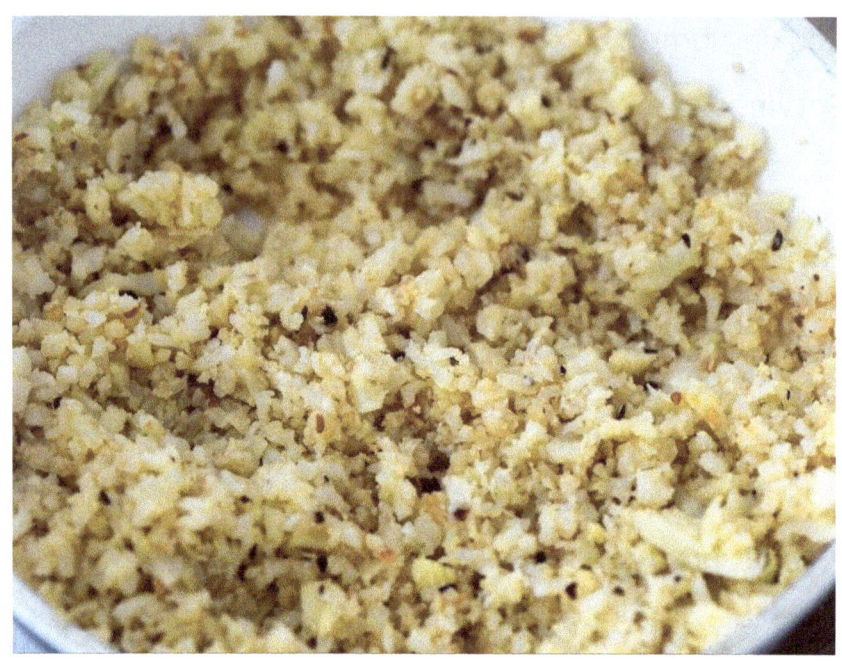

Preparation time: 10 minutes

Cooking time: 15 minutes

Servings: 4

Ingredients:

- 2 tablespoons chia seeds
- 2 cups cauliflower rice

- ½ cup chives, chopped
- ½ cup radishes, halved
- 2 tablespoons avocado oil
- Zest of 1 lime, grated
- 1 cup coconut cream

Directions:

1. Heat up a pan with the oil over medium heat, add the cauliflower rice, chia seeds and the other ingredients, toss, cook for 15 minutes, divide into bowls and serve.

Nutrition:

Calories 220, fat 19.6, fiber 6.9, carbs 10.4, protein 4.1

Creamy Onion Soup

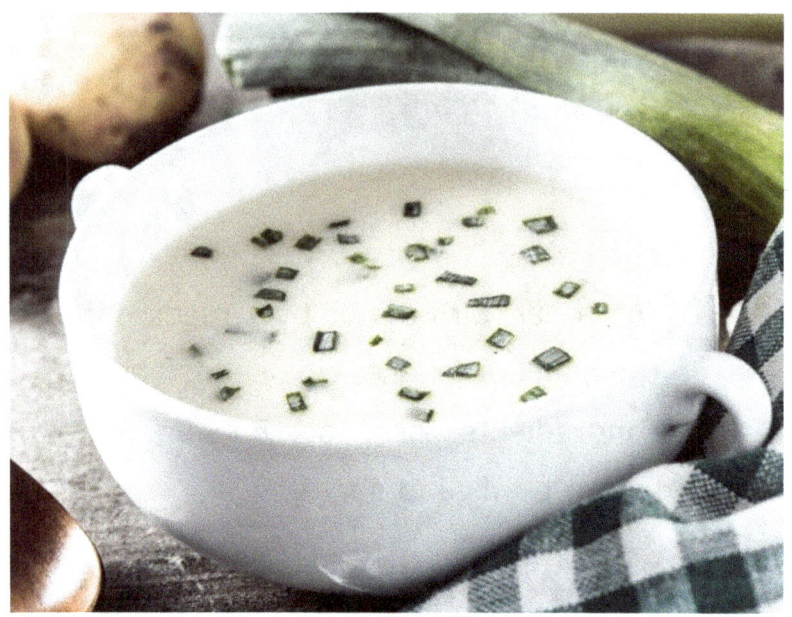

Preparation Time: 15 minutes

Cooking Time: 25 minutes

Servings: 4

Ingredients:

- 1 shallot, sliced
- 1 ½ tablespoons extra-virgin olive oil
- Sea salt

- 1 leek, sliced
- 4 cups vegetable stock
- 1 garlic clove, chopped
- 1 onion, sliced

Directions:

1. Add The Olive Oil And Vegetable Stock Into A Large Saucepan Over Medium Heat, Bring To A Boil.
2. Add The Remaining Ingredients And Stir. Cover And Simmer For 25 Minutes.
3. Puree Your Soup Using A Blender Until Smooth.
4. Serve Warm And Enjoy!

Nutritional Values (Per Serving):

Calories: 90 Sugar: 4.1 G Fat: 7.4 G Carbohydrates: 10.1 G Cholesterol: 0 Mg Protein: 1 G

Creamy Cucumber Egg Salad

Preparation Time: 15 minutes

Servings: 4

Ingredients:

- 1 avocado, peeled, cubed
- 6 eggs, organic, hard-boiled
- 1 medium cucumber, peeled, chopped
- ¼ cup mayonnaise
- ½ teaspoon paprika

Directions:

1. Peel and dice eggs. In a bowl mix ingredients well. Serve and enjoy!

Nutritional Values (Per Serving):

Calories: 176 Fat: 12.7 g Cholesterol: 249 mg Sugar: 2.7 g Carbohydrates: 7.6 g Protein: 9.2 g

Coconut Broccoli Cheese Loaf

Preparation Time: 35 minutes

Servings: 5

Ingredients:

- 5 eggs, lightly beaten
- 3 1/1 tbsp coconut flour
- 2 tsp baking powder
- 3/4 cup broccoli florets, chopped
- 1 cup cheddar cheese, shredded
- 1 tsp salt

Directions:

1. Preheat the oven to 350 °F.
2. Spray a loaf pan with cooking spray and set aside.
3. Add all ingredients into the bowl and mix well.
4. Pour egg mixture into the prepared loaf pan and bake in preheated oven for 30 minutes.
5. Cut loaf into the slices and serve.

Nutritional Value (Amount per Serving):

Calories 209 Fat 13 g Carbohydrates 8 g Sugar 1 g Protein 13 g Cholesterol 187 mg

Creamy Egg Salad

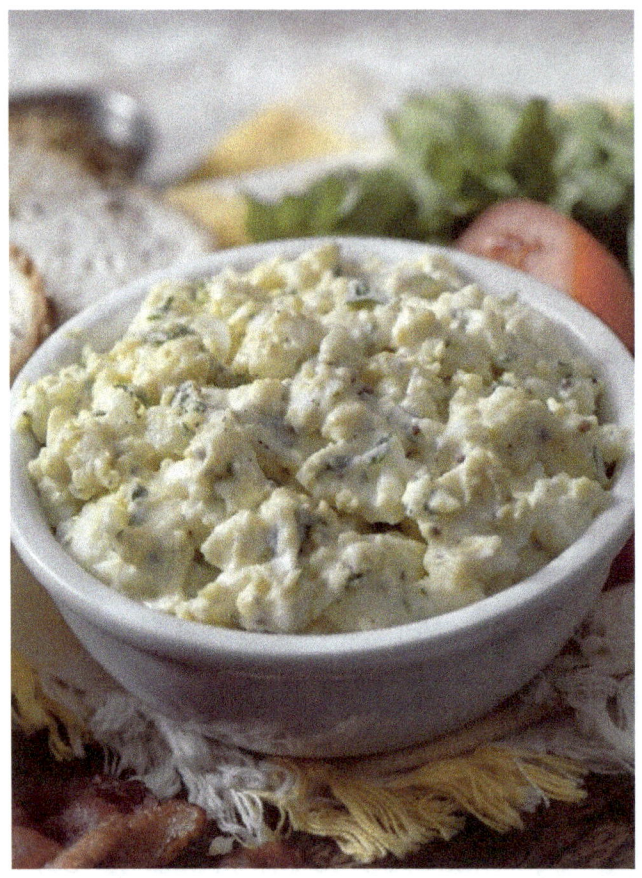

Preparation Time: 15 minutes

Servings: 4

Ingredients:

- 12 eggs, hard-boiled
- 1 scallion, sliced
- 1/2 cup celery, diced
- 3/4 cup mayonnaise
- 1 tbsp Dijon mustard
- Pepper
- Salt

Directions:

1. Separate egg yolks and egg whites.
2. Chop egg whites into small pieces.
3. Add egg yolks, salt, mustard, and mayonnaise in a blender and blend until smooth.
4. Add chopped egg whites, scallion and celery in a large bowl then add egg yolk mixture and mix well.
5. Season with pepper and salt.
6. Serve and enjoy.

Nutritional Value (Amount per Serving):

Calories 367 Fat 28 g Carbohydrates 12 g Sugar 4 g Protein 17 g Cholesterol 503 mg

Avocado Coconut Pie

Preparation Time: 30 minutes

Cooking Time: 50 minutes

Serving: 4

Ingredients:

For the piecrust:

- 1 tbsp flax seed powder + 3 tbsp water
- 4 tbsp chia seeds
- 4 tbsp coconut flour
- ¾ cup almond flour
- 1 tsp baking powder
- 1 tbsp psyllium husk powder
- 1 pinch salt
- 3 tbsp coconut oil
- 4 tbsp water

For the filling:

- 2 ripe avocados
- 1 cup vegan mayonnaise
- 2 tbsp fresh parsley, finely chopped
- 3 tbsp flax seed powder + 9 tbsp water
- 1 jalapeno, finely chopped

- ½ tsp onion powder
- ¼ tsp salt
- ½ cup cashew cream
- 1¼ cups shredded tofu cheese

Directions:

1. In 2 separate bowls, mix the different portions of flax seed powder with the respective quantity of water. Allow absorbing for 5 minutes.
2. Preheat the oven to 350 °F.
3. In a food processor, add the coconut flour, chia seeds, almond flour, psyllium husk powder, baking powder, salt, coconut oil, water, and the smaller portion of the flax egg. Blend the Ingredients until the resulting dough forms into a ball.
4. Line a spring form pan with about 12-inch diameter of parchment paper and spread the dough in the pan. Bake for 10 to 15 minutes or until a light golden brown color is achieved.
5. Meanwhile, cut the avocado into halves lengthwise, remove the pit, and chop the pulp. Put in a bowl and add the mayonnaise, remaining flax egg, parsley, jalapeno, onion

powder, salt, cashew cream, and tofu cheese. Combine well.
6. Remove the piecrust when ready and fill with the creamy mixture. Level the filling with a spatula and continue baking for 35 minutes or until lightly golden brown.
7. When ready, take out. Cool before slicing and serving with a baby spinach salad.

Nutrition:

Calories:680, Total Fat:71.8 g, Saturated Fat:20.9 g, Total Carbs: 10g, Dietary Fiber:7 g, Sugar: 2g, Protein: 3g, Sodium:525 mg

Mushroom Rice

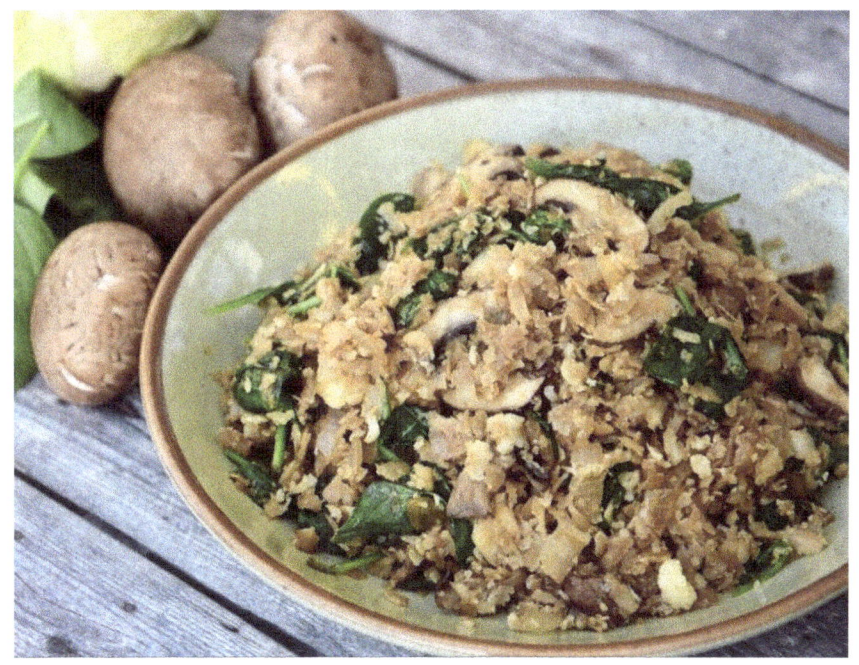

Preparation time: 10 minutes

Cooking time: 20 minutes

Servings: 4

Ingredients:

- 2 tablespoons olive oil
- 1 cup mushrooms, sliced
- 2 cups cauliflower rice

- 2 tablespoons lime juice
- 2 tablespoons almonds, sliced
- 1 cup veggie stock
- ½ teaspoon garlic powder
- Salt and black pepper to the taste
- 1 tablespoon parsley, chopped

Directions:

1. Heat up a pan with the oil over medium heat, add the mushrooms and the almonds and sauté for 5 minutes.
2. Add the cauliflower rice and the other ingredients, toss, cook over medium heat for 15 minutes more, divide between plates and serve.

Nutrition:

Calories 124, fat 2.4, fiber 1.5, carbs 2, protein 1.2

Sage Quinoa

Preparation time: 10 minutes

Cooking time: 30 minutes

Servings: 4

Ingredients:

- 1 tablespoon olive oil
- 1 yellow onion, chopped
- 1 cup quinoa
- 2 cups chicken stock
- 1 tablespoon sage, chopped
- 2 garlic cloves, minced
- A pinch of salt and black pepper
- 1 tablespoon chives, chopped

Directions:

1. Heat up a pan with the oil over medium-high heat, add the onion and the garlic and sauté for 5 minutes.
2. Add the quinoa and the other ingredients, toss, cook over medium heat for 25 minutes more, divide between plates and serve.

Nutrition:

Calories 182, fat 1, fiber 1, carbs 11, protein 8

Mushroom And Peas Risotto

Preparation time: 10 minutes

Cooking time: 1 hour and 30 minutes

Servings: 8

Ingredients:

- 1 shallot, chopped
- 8 ounces white mushrooms, sliced
- 1 and ¾ cup white rice
- 3 tablespoons olive oil
- 1 teaspoon garlic, minced
- 4 cups veggie stock
- 1 cup peas
- Salt and black pepper to the taste

Directions:

1. In your slow cooker, mix oil with shallot, mushrooms, garlic, rice, stock, peas, salt and pepper.
2. Stir, cover and cook on High for 1 hour and 30 minutes.

3. Stir risotto one more time, divide between plates and serve as a side dish.
4. Enjoy!

Nutrition:

Calories 254, fat 7, fiber 3, carbs 27, protein 7

Brussels Sprouts

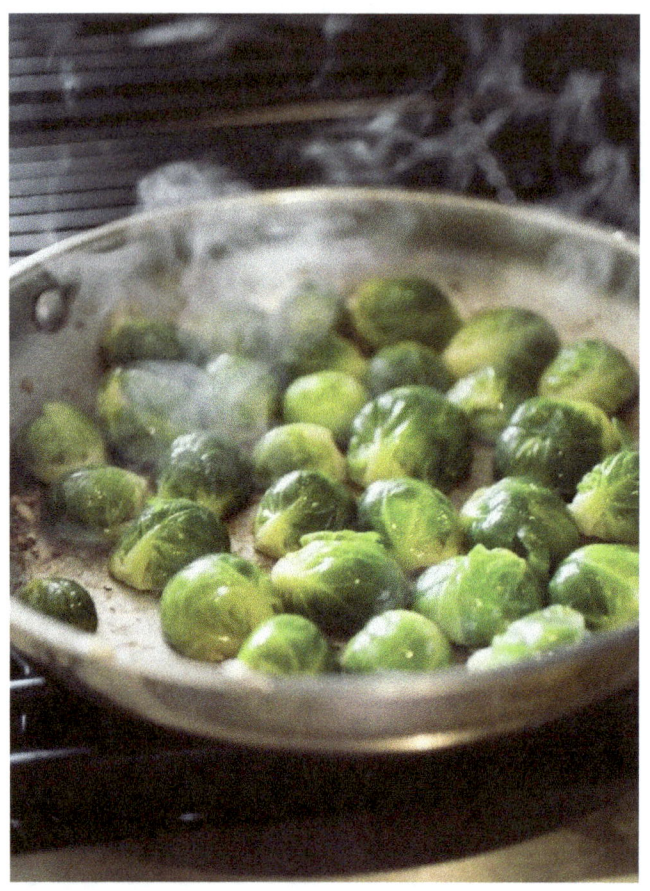

Preparation time: 10 minutes

Cooking time: 3 hours

Servings: 12

Ingredients:

- 1 cup red onion, chopped
- 2 pounds Brussels sprouts, trimmed and halved
- ¼ cup apple juice
- 3 tablespoons olive oil
- ¼ cup maple syrup
- A pinch of salt and black pepper
- 1 tablespoon thyme, chopped

Directions:

1. In your slow cooker, mix Brussels sprouts with onion, salt, pepper and apple juice, toss, cover and cook on Low for 3 hours.
2. In a bowl, mix maple syrup with oil and thyme, whisk really well and add over Brussels sprouts.
3. Toss well, divide between plates and serve as a side dish.
4. Enjoy!

Nutrition:

Calories 100, fat 4, fiber 4, carbs 14, protein 3

Italian Veggie Side Dish

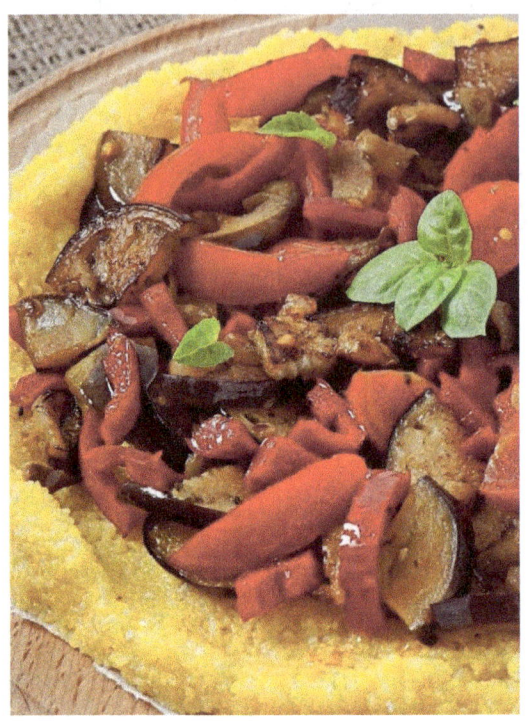

Preparation time: 10 minutes

Cooking time: 6 hours

Servings: 8

Ingredients:

- 38 ounces canned cannellini beans, drained
- 19 ounces canned fava beans, drained

- ¼ cup basil pesto
- 1 yellow onion, chopped
- 4 garlic cloves, minced
- 1 and ½ teaspoon Italian seasoning, dried and crushed
- 1 tomato, chopped
- 15 ounces already cooked polenta, cut into medium pieces
- 2 cups spinach
- 1 cup radicchio, torn

Directions:

1. In your slow cooker, mix cannellini beans with fava beans, basil pesto, onion, garlic, Italian seasoning, polenta, tomato, spinach and radicchio, toss, cover and cook on Low for 6 hours.
2. Divide between plates and serve as a side dish.
3. Enjoy!

Nutrition:

Calories 364, fat 12, fiber 10, carbs 45, protein 21

Roasted Artichokes and Sauce

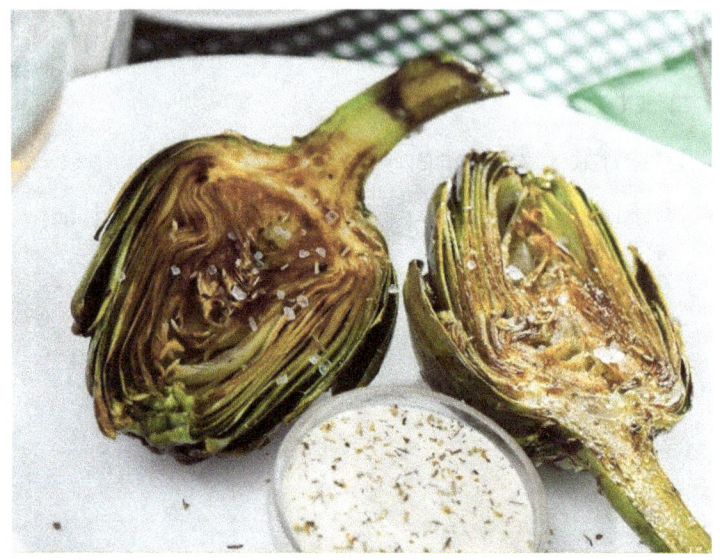

Preparation time: 10 minutes

Cooking time: 30 minutes

Servings: 4

Ingredients:
- 2 big artichokes, trimmed and halved
- Juice of 1 lime
- 2 tablespoons avocado oil
- 1 teaspoon turmeric powder

- 1 cup coconut cream
- ½ teaspoon onion powder
- ¼ teaspoon sweet paprika
- A pinch of salt and black pepper
- 1 teaspoon cumin, ground

Directions:

1. In a roasting pan, combine the artichokes with the oil, the lime juice and the other ingredients, toss and bake at 390 degrees F for 30 minutes.
2. Divide the artichokes and sauce between plates and serve.

Nutrition:

Calories 190, fat 6, fiber 8, carbs 10, protein 9

Sage Pecan Cauliflower

Preparation Time: 10 minutes

Cooking Time: 30 minutes

Servings: 6

Ingredients:

- 1 large cauliflower head, cut into florets
- 1/2 tsp dried thyme
- 1/2 tsp poultry seasoning
- 1/4 cup olive oil
- 1/4 cup pecans, chopped
- 2 tbsp parsley, chopped
- 2 garlic clove, minced
- 1/2 tsp ground sage
- 1/4 cup celery, chopped
- 1 onion, sliced
- 1/4 tsp black pepper
- 1 tsp sea salt

Directions:

1. Preheat the oven to 450 °F/ 232 °C.
2. Spray a baking tray with cooking spray and set

aside.
3. In a large bowl, mix together cauliflower, thyme, poultry seasoning, olive oil, garlic, celery, sage, onions, pepper, and salt.
4. Spread mixture on a baking tray and roast in preheated oven for 15 minutes.
5. Add pecans and parsley and stir well. Roast for 10-15 minutes more.
6. Serve and enjoy.

nutrition:

Calories 118, Fat 8.6g, Carbohydrates 9.9g, Sugar 4.2g, Protein 3.1g, Cholesterol 0mg

Ratatouille (Pressure cooker)

Preparation time: 15 minutes

Servings: 4-6

Ingredients

- 1 onion, diced
- 3 or 4 tomatoes, diced
- 1 eggplant, cubed
- 4 garlic cloves, minced
- 1 to 2 teaspoons olive oil
- 1 cup water
- 1 or 2 bell peppers, any color, seeded and chopped
- 1½ tablespoons dried herbes de Provence (or any mixture of dried basil, oregano, thyme, marjoram, and rosemary
- ½ teaspoon salt
- Freshly ground black pepper

Directions

1. On your electric pressure cooker, select Sauté. Add the onion, garlic, and olive oil. Cook for 4 to

5 minutes, stirring occasionally, until the onion is softened. Add the water, tomatoes, eggplant, bell peppers, and herbes de Provence. Cancel Sauté.

2. High pressure for 6 minutes. Close and lock the lid, ensure the pressure valve is sealed, select High Pressure, and set the time for 6 minutes.

3. Pressure Release. Once the cook time is complete, let the pressure release naturally, about 20 minutes. Once all the pressure has released, carefully unlock and remove the lid. Let cool for a few minutes, then season with salt and pepper.

Nutrition

Calories: 101; Total fat: 2g; Protein: 4g; Sodium: 304mg; Fiber: 7g

Creamy Garlic-Spinach Rotini Soup

Preparation time: 10 minutes

cooking time: 15 minutes

servings: 4

Ingredients

- 1 teaspoon olive oil
- 2 peeled carrots or ½ red bell pepper, chopped
- 1 cup chopped mushrooms
- 4 garlic cloves, minced, or 1 teaspoon garlic powder
- ¼ teaspoon plus a pinch salt
- 6 cups Economical Vegetable Broth or water
- Pinch freshly ground black pepper
- 1 cup rotini or gnocchi
- ¾ cup unsweetened nondairy milk
- ¼ cup nutritional yeast
- 2 cups chopped fresh spinach
- ¼ cup pitted black olives or sun-dried tomatoes, chopped
- Herbed Croutons, for topping (optional)

Directions

1. Heat the olive oil in a large soup pot over medium-high heat.
2. Add the mushrooms and a pinch of salt. Sauté for about 4 minutes, until the mushrooms are softened. Add the garlic (if using fresh) and carrots, sauté for 1 minute more.
3. Add the vegetable broth, remaining ¼ teaspoon of salt, and pepper (plus the garlic powder, if using).
4. Bring to a boil and add the pasta. Cook for about 10 minutes, until the pasta is just cooked.
5. Turn off the heat and stir in the milk, nutritional yeast, spinach, and olives. Top with croutons (if using).
6. Leftovers will keep in an airtight container for up to 1 week in the refrigerator or up to 1 month in the freezer.

Nutrition (2 cups)

Calories: 207; Protein: 11g; Total fat: 5g; Saturated fat: 1g; Carbohydrates: 34g; Fiber: 7g

Italian Wedding Soup

Preparation time: 10 minutes

cooking time: 15 minutes

servings: 4

Ingredients

- 1 teaspoon olive oil
- 2 carrots, peeled and chopped
- ½ onion, chopped
- 3 or 4 garlic cloves, minced, or ½ teaspoon garlic powder
- 8 cups water or Economical Vegetable Broth
- 1 cup orzo or pearl couscous
- 1 tablespoon dried herbs
- 2 cups chopped greens, such as spinach, kale, or chard
- Freshly ground black pepper
- 1 recipe quinoa meatballs
- Salt

Directions

1. Heat the olive oil in a large soup pot over medium-high heat.
2. Add the carrots, onion, garlic (if using fresh), and a pinch of salt. Sauté for 3 to 4 minutes, until softened. Add the water, orzo, and dried herbs (plus the garlic powder, if using).
3. Season to taste with salt and pepper, and bring the soup to a boil. Turn the heat to low and simmer until the orzo is soft, about 10 minutes.
4. Add the meatballs and greens, and stir until the greens are wilted.
5. Taste and season with more salt and pepper as needed.
6. Leftovers will keep in an airtight container for up to 1 week in the refrigerator or up to 1 month in the freezer.

Nutrition (2 cups)

Calories: 168; Protein: 9g; Total fat: 3g; Saturated fat: 0g; Carbohydrates: 30g; Fiber: 6g

Tomato Orzo Soup

Preparation time: 5 minutes

cooking time: 30 minutes

servings: 4

Ingredients

- 1 tablespoon olive oil
- 1 medium onion, chopped
- 1 celery rib, minced
- 3 garlic cloves, minced
- 1 (28-ouncecan crushed tomatoes
- 3 cups chopped fresh ripe tomatoes
- 2 bay leaves
- 2 tablespoons tomato paste
- 3 cups vegetable broth, homemade (see Light Vegetable Broth or store-bought, or water
- Salt and freshly ground black pepper
- 1 cup plain unsweetened soy milk
- 11/2 cups cooked orzo
- 2 tablespoons chopped fresh basil, for garnish

Directions

1. In large soup pot, heat the oil over medium heat. Add the onion, celery, and garlic. Cover and cook until softened, about 5 minutes. Stir in the canned and fresh tomatoes, tomato paste, broth, sugar, and bay leaves. Season with salt and pepper to taste and bring to a boil. Reduce the heat to low, cover, and simmer, uncovered, until the vegetables are tender, about 20 minutes.
2. Remove and discard bay leaves. Puree the soup in the pot with an immersion blender or in a blender or food processor, in batches if necessary, and return to the pot. Stir in the soy milk, taste, adjusting seasonings if necessary, and heat through.
3. Spoon about 1/3 cup of the orzo into the bottom of each bowl, ladle the hot soup on top, and serve sprinkled with the basil.

Golden Potato Soup

Preparation time: 5 minutes

cooking time: 30 minutes

servings: 4 to 6

Ingredients

- 1 tablespoon olive oil3 medium shallots, chopped4 cups vegetable broth, homemade (see Light Vegetable Broth or store-bought, or water
- 1 cup plain unsweetened soy milk
- 2 medium sweet potatoes, peeled and diced
- 3 medium russet potatoes, peeled and diced
- Salt and freshly ground black pepper
- 1 tablespoon minced chives, for garnish

Directions

1. In large saucepan, heat the oil over medium heat. Add the shallots, cover, and cook until softened, about 5 minutes.
2. Add the broth and potatoes and bring to a boil.

3. Reduce heat to low and simmer, uncovered, until the potatoes are soft, about 20 minutes.
4. Puree the potato mixture in the pot with an immersion blender or in a blender or food processor, in batches if necessary, and return to the pot.
5. Stir in the soy milk and season with salt and pepper to taste.
6. Simmer for 5 minutes to heat through and blend flavors.
7. Ladle the soup into bowls, sprinkle with chives, and serve.

Coconut and Curry Soup

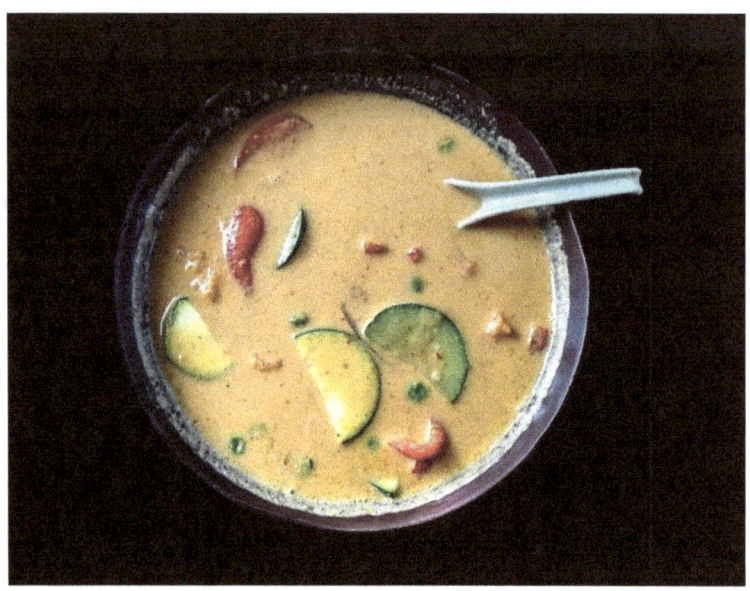

Preparation Time: 15 Minutes

Cooking Time: 15 Minutes

Servings: 4

Ingredients

- 1 carrot, peeled and julienned
- 1 tablespoon coconut oil
- ½ onion, thinly sliced
- ½ cup sliced shiitake mushrooms

- juice from 1 lime, or 2 teaspoons lime juice
- 3 garlic cloves, minced
- one 14-ounce can coconut milk
- 1 cup vegetable stock
- ½ teaspoon sea salt
- 2 teaspoons curry powder

Directions

1. Preparing the Ingredients
2. In a large soup pot, heat the coconut oil over medium-high heat until it shimmers.
3. Add the onion, carrot, and mushrooms and cook until soft, about 7 minutes.
4. Stir in the garlic and cook until it is fragrant, about 30 seconds.
5. Add the coconut milk, vegetable stock, lime juice, salt, and curry powder and heat through.
6. Serve immediately.

Spicy Black Bean Orzo Soup

Preparation Time: 5 Minutes

Cooking Time: 50 Minutes

Servings: 4 To 6

Ingredients

- 2 tablespoons olive oil
- 3 garlic cloves, minced
- 1 tablespoon chili powder
- 4 1/2 cups cooked or 3 (15.5-ounce) cans black beans, drained and rinsed
- 1 teaspoon dried oregano
- 1 small jalapeño, seeded and finely chopped (optional)
- 1/4 cup minced oil-packed sun-dried tomatoes
- 4 cups vegetable broth, homemade (see Light Vegetable Broth) or store-bought, or water
- 1 cup water
- Salt and freshly ground black pepper
- 1/2 cup orzo
- 2 tablespoons chopped fresh cilantro, for garnish

Directions

1. In a large soup pot, heat the oil over medium heat. Add the garlic and cook until fragrant, about 1 minute. Stir in the chili powder, oregano, beans, jalapeño, if using, tomatoes, broth, water, and salt and pepper to taste. Simmer for 30 minutes to blend flavors.
2. Puree the soup in the pot with an immersion blender or in a blender or food processor, in batches if necessary, and return to the pot. Cook the soup 15 minutes longer over medium heat. Taste, adjusting seasonings, and add more water if necessary.
3. While the soup is simmering, cook the orzo in a pot of boiling salted water, stirring occasionally, until al dente, about 5 minutes. Drain the orzo and divide it among the soup bowls. Ladle the soup into the bowls, garnish with cilantro, and serve.

Minestrone

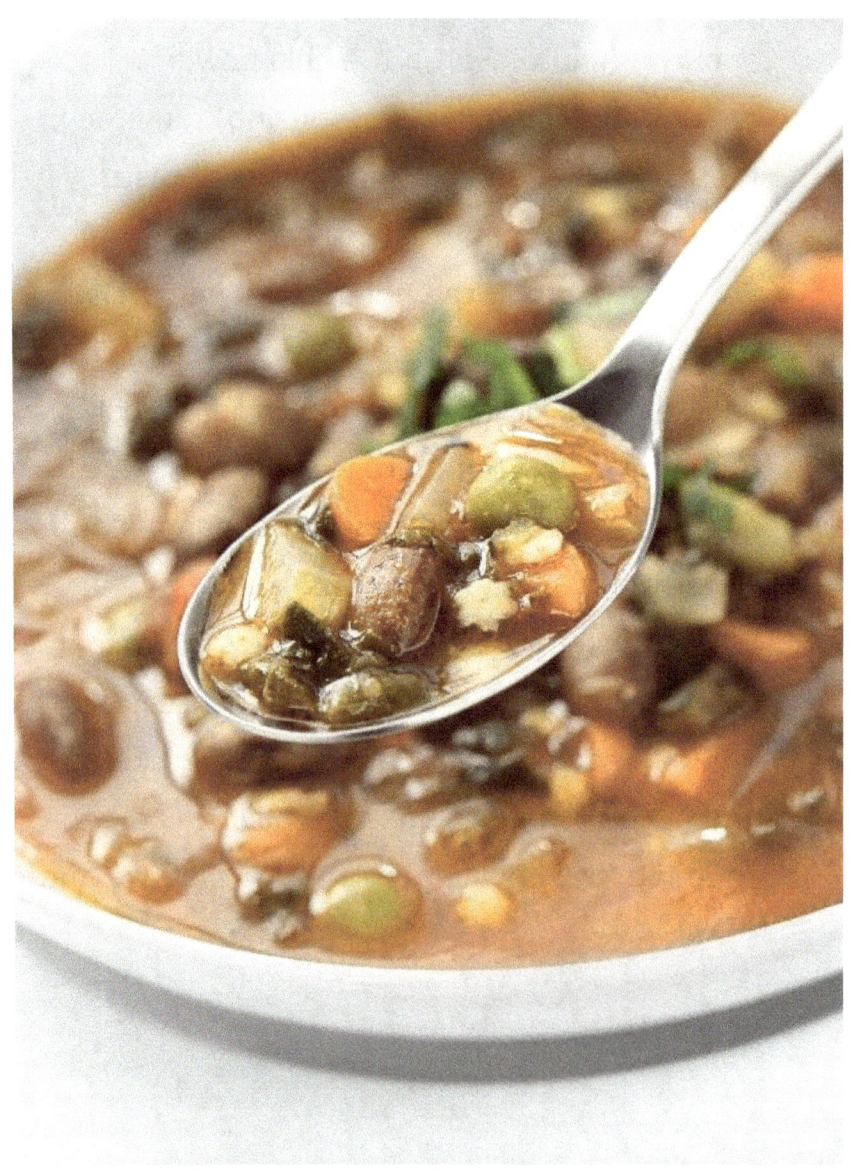

Preparation Time: 15 Minutes

Cooking Time: 15 Minutes

Servings:4

Ingredients

- 2 tablespoons olive oil
- ½ onion, diced
- 1 zucchini, diced
- 1 carrot, peeled and diced
- 1 stalk celery, diced
- 4 garlic cloves, minced
- 5 cups vegetable stock
- one 15-ounce can kidney beans, drained and rinsed
- one 15-ounce can chopped tomatoes with liquid, or 2 fresh tomatoes, peeled and chopped
- 2 teaspoons italian seasoning
- sea salt
- freshly ground pepper

Directions

1. In a large soup pot, heat the olive oil over medium-high heat until it shimmers.

2. Add the onion, carrot, and celery and cook until vegetables soften, about 5 minutes.
3. Add the garlic and cook until it is fragrant, about 30 seconds.
4. Add the vegetable stock, zucchini, kidney beans, tomatoes, and Italian seasoning.
5. Simmer the soup until the vegetables are soft, about 10 minutes.
6. Season with salt and pepper and serve immediately.

Black And Gold Gazpacho

Preparation Time: 15 Minutes

Cooking Time: 0 Minutes

Servings: 4

Ingredients

- 1 1/2 pounds ripe yellow tomatoes, chopped
- 1 large cucumber, peeled, seeded, and chopped
- 1 large yellow bell pepper, seeded, and chopped
- 4 green onions, white part only
- 2 tablespoons white wine vinegar
- 2 garlic cloves, minced
- 2 tablespoons olive oil
- Ground cayenne
- 1 1/2 cups cooked or 1 (15.5-ounce) can black beans, drained and rinsed
- 2 tablespoons minced fresh parsley
- Salt
- 1 cup toasted croutons (optional)

Directions

1. In a blender or food processor, combine half the tomatoes with the cucumber, bell pepper, green onions, and garlic. Process until smooth. Add the oil and vinegar, season with salt and cayenne to taste, and process until blended.
2. Transfer the soup to a large nonmetallic bowl and stir in the black beans and remaining tomatoes. Cover the bowl and refrigerate for 1 to 2 hours. Taste, adjusting seasonings if necessary.
3. Ladle the soup into bowls, garnish with parsley and croutons, if using, and serve.

Parsley-Lime Pasta

Preparation Time: 20 minutes

Serving: 4

Ingredients:

- 2 tbsp butter
- 1 lb tempeh, chopped
- 1 lime, zested and juiced
- 4 garlic cloves, minced
- 1 pinch red chili flakes
- ¼ cup white wine
- 3 medium zucchinis, spiralized
- Salt and black pepper to taste
- 2 tbsp chopped parsley
- 1 cup grated parmesan cheese for topping

Directions:

1. Melt the butter in a large skillet and cook in the tempeh until golden brown.
2. Flip and stir in the garlic and red chili flakes. Cook further for 1 minute; transfer to a plate and set aside.

3. Pour the wine and lime juice into the skillet, and cook until reduced by a quarter. Meanwhile, stir to deglaze the bottom of the pot.
4. Mix in the zucchinis, lime zest, tempeh and parsley. Season with salt and black pepper, and toss everything well. Cook until the zucchinis is slightly tender for 2 minutes.
5. Dish the food onto serving plates and top generously with the parmesan cheese.

Nutrition:

Calories: 326, Total Fat: 24.9g, Saturated Fat:12.9 g, Total Carbs: 6 g, Dietary Fiber:1g, Sugar: 4g, Protein: 20g, Sodium: 568mg

Creamy Seitan Shirataki Fettucine

Preparation Time: 35 minutes

Serving: 4

Ingredients:

For the shirataki fettuccine:

- 2 (8 oz) packs shirataki fettuccine

For the creamy seitan sauce:

- 5 tbsp butter
- 4 seitan slabs, cut into 2-inch cubes
- 3 garlic cloves, minced
- 1 ¼ cups coconut cream
- ½ cup dry white wine
- 1 tsp grated lemon zest
- 1 cup baby spinach
- Salt and black pepper to taste
- Lemon wedges for garnishing

Directions:

For the shirataki fettuccine:

1. Boil 2 cups of water in a medium pot over medium heat.
2. Strain the shirataki pasta through a colander and rinse very well under hot running water.
3. Allow proper draining and pour the shirataki pasta into the boiling water. Cook for 3 minutes and strain again.
4. Place a dry skillet over medium heat and stir-fry the shirataki pasta until visibly dry, and makes a squeaky sound when stirred, 1 to 2 minutes.
5. Take off the heat and set aside.

For the seitan sauce:

6. Melt half of the butter in a large skillet; season the seitan with salt, black pepper, and cook in the butter until golden brown on all sides and flaky within, 8 minutes.
7. Transfer to a plate and set aside.
8. Add the remaining butter to the skillet to melt and stir in the garlic. Cook until fragrant, 1 minute.

9. Mix in the coconut cream, white wine, lemon zest, salt, and black pepper. Allow boiling over low heat until the sauce thickens, 5 minutes.
10. Stir in the spinach, allow wilting for 2 minutes and stir in the shirataki fettuccine and seitan until well-coated in the sauce. Adjust the taste with salt and black pepper.
11. Dish the food and garnish with the lemon wedges. Serve warm.

Nutrition:

Calories: 720, Total Fat: 56.5g, Saturated Fat: 27.2g, Total Carbs: 17 g, Dietary Fiber:3g, Sugar: 7g, Protein: 37g, Sodium:1764 mg

Tomato Avocado Cucumber Salad

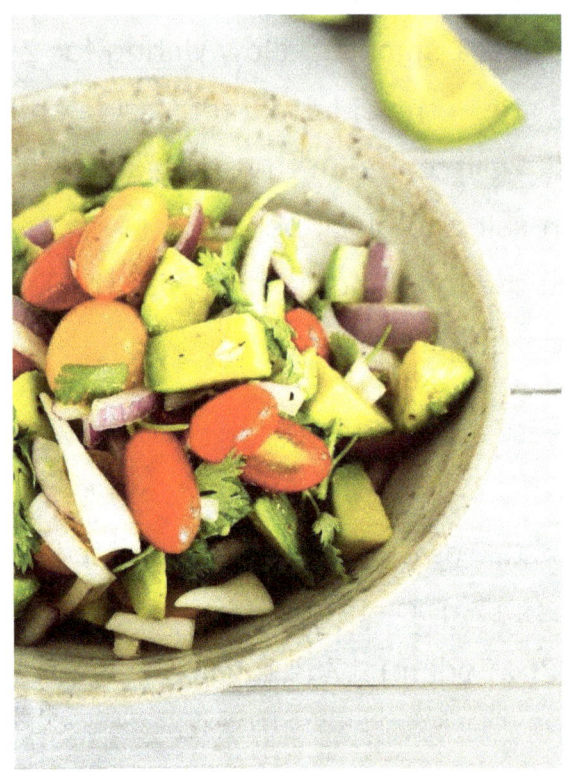

Preparation Time: 10 minutes

Cooking Time: 0 minutes

Serves: 4

Ingredients:

- 1 cucumber, sliced

- ½ onion, sliced
- avocado, chopped
- tomatoes, chopped
- 1 bell pepper, chopped

For Dressings:

- tbsp cilantro
- ¼ tsp garlic powder
- tbsp olive oil
- ½ tsp black pepper
- 1 tbsp lemon juice
- ½ tsp salt

Directions:

1. In a small bowl, mix together all dressing ingredients and set aside.
2. Add all salad ingredients into the large mixing bowl and mix well.
3. Pour dressing over salad and toss well.
4. Serve immediately and enjoy.

nutrition:

Calories 130 Fat 9.8 g Carbohydrates 10.6 g Sugar 5.1 g Protein 2.1 g Cholesterol 0 mg

Avocado Almond Cabbage Salad

Preparation Time: 15 minutes

Cooking Time: 0 minutes

Servings: 3

Ingredients:

- 3 cups savoy cabbage, shredded
- 1 avocado, chopped
- cup ½ blanched almonds
- ¼ tsp pepper
- ¼ tsp sea salt

For Dressings:

- 1 tsp coconut aminos
- ½ tsp Dijon mustard
- 1 tbsp lemon juice
- 3 tbsp olive oil
- Pepper
- Salt

Directions:

1. In a small bowl, mix together all dressing ingredients and set aside.

2. Add all salad ingredients to the large bowl and mix well.
3. Pour dressing over salad and toss well.
4. Serve immediately and enjoy.

nutrition:

Calories 317 Fat 14.1 g Carbohydrates 39.8 g Sugar 9.3 g Protein 11.6 g Cholesterol 0 mg

Rich Chickpeas And Lentils Soup

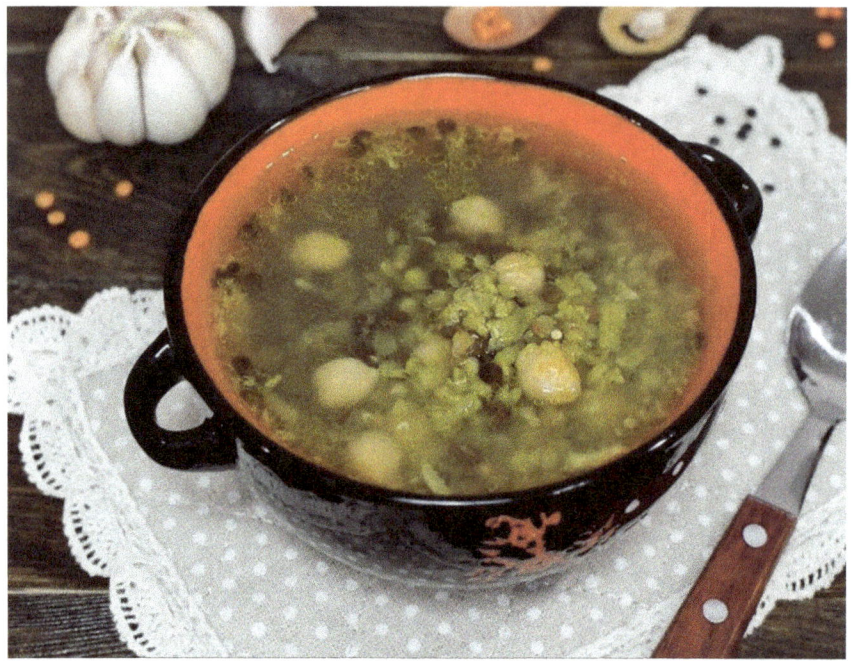

Preparation time: 10 minutes

Cooking time: 5 hours

Servings: 6

Ingredients:

- 1 yellow onion, chopped
- 1 tablespoon garlic, minced
- 1 tablespoon olive oil

- 29 ounces canned tomatoes and juice
- 1 teaspoons sweet paprika
- 1 teaspoon smoked paprika
- 1 cup red lentils
- 15 ounces canned chickpeas, drained
- 4 cups veggie stock
- Salt and black pepper to the taste

Directions:

1. In your slow cooker, mix onion with oil, garlic, sweet and smoked paprika, salt, pepper, lentils, chickpeas, stock and tomatoes, stir, cover and cook on High for 5 hours.
2. Ladle into bowls and serve hot.
3. Enjoy!

nutrition:

Calories 341, fat 5, fiber 8, carbs 19, protein 3

Not-Tuna Salad

Preparation time: 5 minutes

cooking time: 0 minutes

servings: 4

Ingredients

- 1 (15.5-ouncecan chickpeas, drained and rinsed
- ½ cup chopped yellow or white onion
- 1 (14-ouncecan hearts of palm, drained and chopped
- ½ cup diced celery
- ¼ cup vegan mayonnaise, plus more if needed
- ½ teaspoon salt
- ¼ teaspoon freshly ground black pepper

Directions

1. In a medium bowl, use a potato masher or fork to roughly mash the chickpeas until chunky and "shredded." Add the hearts of palm, onion, celery, vegan mayonnaise, salt, and pepper.

2. Combine and add more mayonnaise, if necessary, for a creamy texture. Into each of 4 single-serving containers, place ¾ cup of salad. Seal the lids.

Nutrition:

Calories: 214; Fat: 6g; Protein: 9g; Carbohydrates: 35g; Fiber: 8g; Sugar: 1g; Sodium: 765mg

Red Bean and Corn Salad

Preparation time: 15 minutes

cooking time: 0 minutes

servings: 4

Ingredients

- ¼ cup Cashew Cream or other salad dressing
- 2 cups frozen corn, thawed, or 2 cups canned corn, drained
- 1 teaspoon chili powder
- 2 (14.5-ouncecans kidney beans, rinsed and drained
- 1 cup cooked farro, barley, or rice (optional)
- 8 cups chopped romaine lettuce

Directions

1. Line up 4 wide-mouth glass quart jars.
2. In a small bowl, whisk the cream and chili powder.
3. Pour 1 tablespoon of cream into each jar. In each jar, add ¾ cup kidney beans, ½ cup corn, ¼ cup cooked farro (if using), and 2 cups

romaine, punching it down to fit it into the jar. Close the lids tightly.

Nutrition:

Calories: 303; Fat: 9g; Protein: 14g; Carbohydrates: 45g; Fiber: 15g; Sugar: 6g; Sodium: 654mg

Roasted Beet and Avocado Salad

Preparation time: 10 minutes

cooking time: 30minutes

servings: 2

Ingredients

- 2 beets, peeled and thinly sliced
- 1 avocado
- 1 teaspoon olive oil
- Pinch sea salt
- 2 cups mixed greens
- 3 to 4 tablespoons Creamy Balsamic Dressing
- 2 tablespoons chopped almonds, pumpkin seeds, or sunflower seeds (raw or toasted

Directions

1. Preheat the oven to 400 °F.
2. Put the beets, oil, and salt in a large bowl, and toss the beets with your hands to coat.
3. Lay them in a single layer in a large baking dish, and roast them in the oven 20 to 30 minutes, or until they're softened and slightly browned

around the edges.
4. While the beets are roasting, cut the avocado in half and take the pit out.
5. Scoop the flesh out, as intact as possible, and slice it into crescents.
6. Once the beets are cooked, lay slices out on two plates and top each beet slice with a similar-size avocado slice.
7. Top with a handful of mixed greens.
8. Drizzle the dressing over everything, and sprinkle on a few chopped almonds.

Nutrition

Calories: 167; Total fat: 13g; Carbs: 15g; Fiber: 5g; Protein: 4g

Deconstructed Hummus Pitas

Preparation time: 15 minutes

cooking time: 0 minutes

servings: 4 pitas

Ingredients

- 1 garlic clove, crushed
- ¾ cup tahini (sesame paste
- 1/4 cup water
- 2 tablespoons fresh lemon juice
- 1 teaspoon salt
- 1/8 teaspoon ground cayenne
- 11/2 cups cooked or 1 (15.5-ouncecan chickpeas, rinsed and drained
- 2 medium carrots, grated (about 1 cup
- 4 (7-inchpita breads, preferably whole wheat, halved
- 1 large ripe tomato, cut into 1/4-inch slices
- 2 cups fresh baby spinach

Directions

1. In a blender or food processor, mince the garlic. Add the tahini, lemon juice, salt, cayenne, and water. Process until smooth.
2. Place the chickpeas in a bowl and crush slightly with a fork. Add the carrots and the reserved tahini sauce and toss to combine. Set aside.
3. Spoon 2 or 3 tablespoons of the chickpea mixture into each pita half. Tuck a tomato slice and a few spinach leaves into each pocket and serve.

Mushroom Cakes

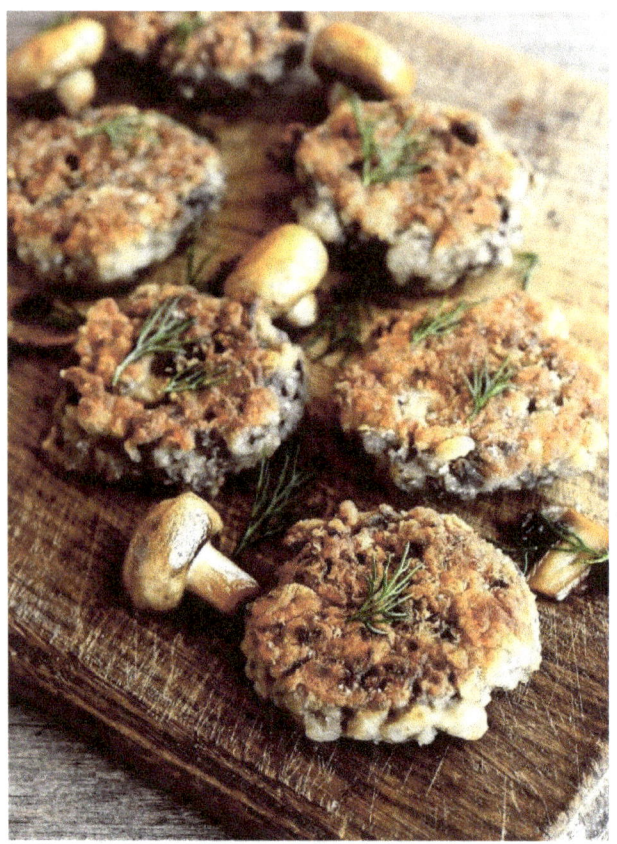

Preparation time: 10 minutes

Cooking time: 12 minutes

Servings: 6

Ingredients:

- 1 cup shallots, chopped
- 2 tablespoons olive oil
- 1 pound mushrooms, minced
- 3 garlic cloves, minced
- 2 tablespoons almond flour
- ¼ cup coconut cream
- 1 tablespoon flaxseed mixed with 2 tablespoons water
- ¼ cup parsley, chopped

Directions:

1. In a bowl, combine the shallots with the garlic, the mushrooms and the other ingredients except the oil, stir well and shape medium cakes out of this mix.
2. Heat up a pan with the oil over medium heat, add the mushroom cakes, cook for 6 minutes on each side, arrange them on a platter and serve as an appetizer.

Nutrition:

Calories 222, fat 4, fiber 3, carbs 8, protein 10

Arugula Dip

Preparation time: 10 minutes

Cooking time: 0 minutes

Servings: 4

Ingredients:

- ½ cup coconut cream
- 2 cups baby arugula
- 2 tablespoons walnuts, chopped
- 2 tablespoons olive oil
- A pinch of salt and black pepper
- Juice of 1 lime
- 2 garlic cloves minced
- ¼ teaspoon red pepper flakes, crushed

Directions:

1. In a blender, combine the arugula with the cream, lime juice and the other ingredients, pulse well, divide into bowls and serve as a party dip.

Nutrition:

Calories 100, fat 0, fiber 1, carbs 1, protein 3

Basil Eggplant Tapenade

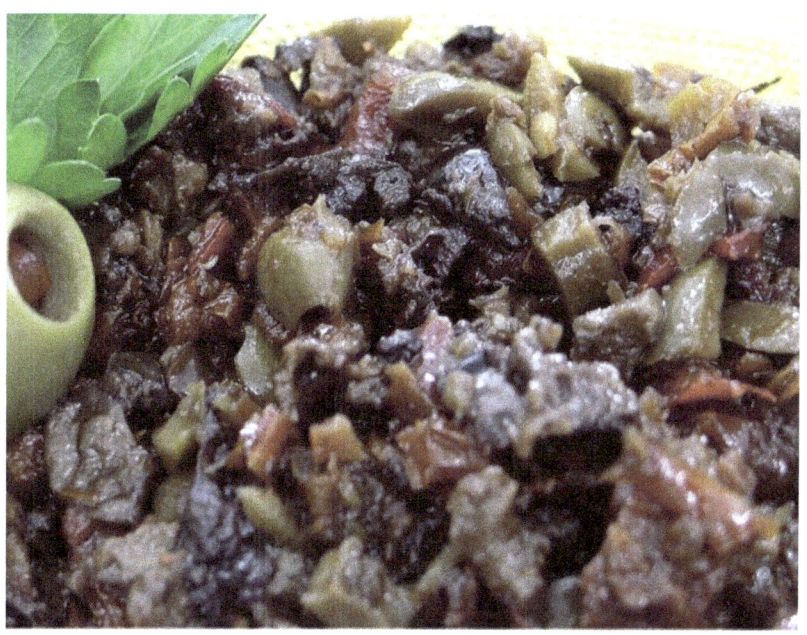

Preparation time: 10 minutes

Cooking time: 15 minutes

Servings: 4

Ingredients:

- 2 eggplants, cubed
- 1 cup cherry tomatoes, cubed
- 2 tablespoons kalamata olives, pitted and cubed

- 3 garlic cloves, minced
- 1 avocado, peeled, pitted and cubed
- 2 tablespoons olive oil
- 2 teaspoons balsamic vinegar
- 1 tablespoon basil, chopped
- A pinch of salt and black pepper

Directions:

1. Heat up a pan with the oil over medium heat, add the garlic, salt and pepper and sauté for 2 minutes.
2. Add the tomatoes, eggplants and the other ingredients, toss, cook over medium heat for 13 minutes, divide into small bowls and serve as an appetizer.

Nutrition:

Calories 121, fat 3, fiber 1, carbs 8, protein 12

Green Beans Dip

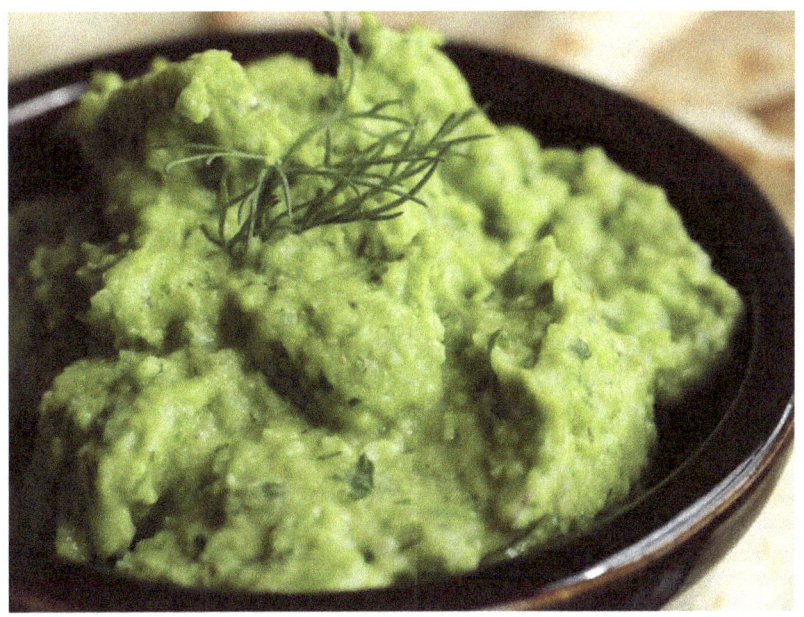

Preparation time: 10 minutes

Cooking time: 25 minutes

Servings: 4

Ingredients:

- 1 pound green beans, trimmed and halved
- 1 teaspoon turmeric powder
- 4 scallions, chopped
- 3 garlic cloves, minced

- 1 teaspoon rosemary, dried
- 1 and ½ cups coconut cream
- 1 tablespoon chives, chopped
- A pinch of salt and black pepper

Directions:

1. In a pan, combine the green beans with the scallions, turmeric and the other ingredients, stir, cook over medium heat for 25 minutes and transfer to a bowl.
2. Blend the mix well, divide into bowls and serve as a party dip.

Nutrition:

Calories 172, fat 6, fiber 3, carbs 6, protein 8

Brussels sprouts Chips

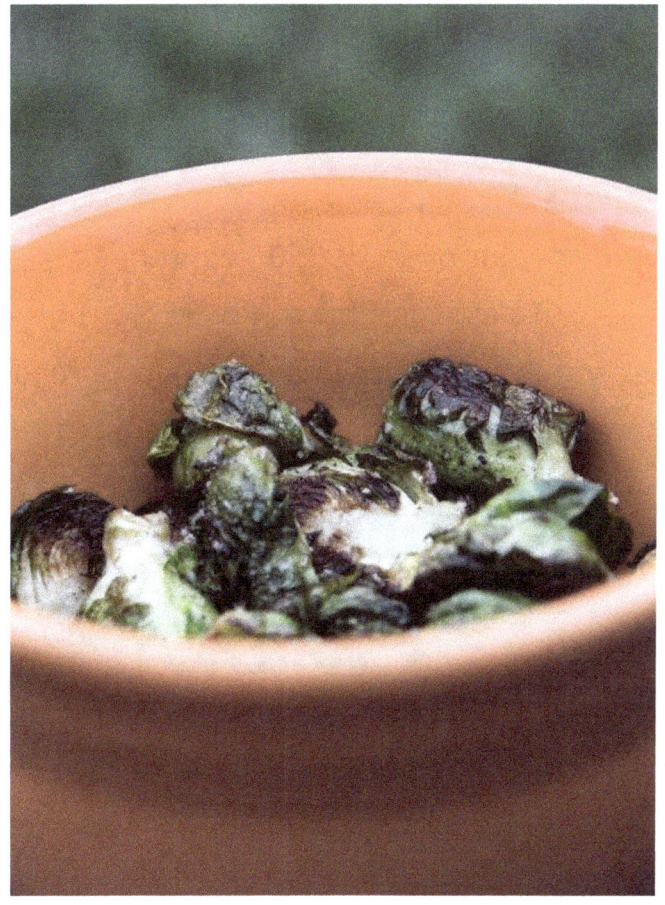

Preparation Time: 10 minutes

Cooking Time: 10 minutes

Servings: 2

Ingredients

- 10 Brussels sprouts split leaves
- 1 tbsp. olive oil
- ¼ tsp. sea salt

Directions:

1. Preheat your oven to 350° Fahrenheit.
2. Toss Brussels sprouts with olive oil.
3. Season Brussels sprouts with salt. Spread Brussels sprouts in a baking dish and bake in preheated oven for 10 minutes.
4. Serve and enjoy!

Nutrition:

Calories: 101, Fat: 7.3g, Cabs: 8.6g, Protein: 3.2g

Quinoa and Black Bean Burgers

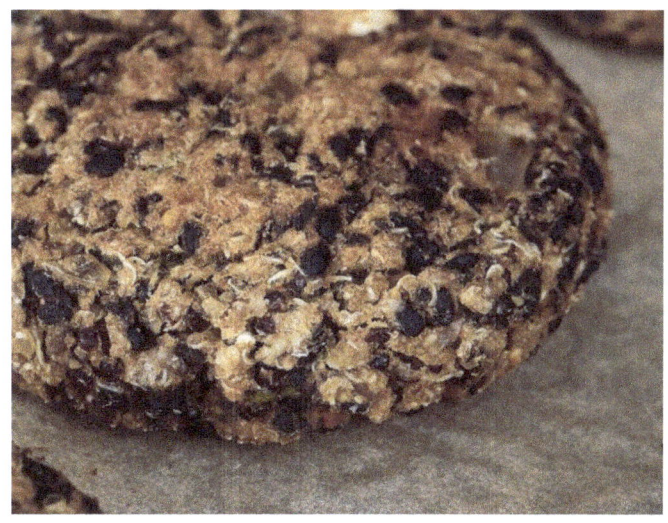

Preparation Time: 10 minutes

Cooking Time: 6 minutes

Servings: 5

Ingredients:

- 1/4 cup quinoa, cooked
- 15 ounces cooked black beans
- 1/4 cup minced bell pepper
- 2 tablespoons minced white onion
- ½ teaspoon minced garlic

- 1/2 cup breadcrumbs
- 1/2 teaspoon salt
- 1 1/2 teaspoons ground cumin
- 1 teaspoon hot pepper sauce
- 3 tablespoons olive oil
- 1 flax egg

Directions:

1. Place all the ingredients in a bowl, except for oil, stir until well combined, and then shape the mixture into five patties.
2. Heat oil in a frying pan over medium heat, add patties and cook for 3 minutes per side until browned.
3. Serve straight away.

Nutrition:

Calories: 245 Cal, Fat: 10.6 g, Carbs: 29 g, Protein: 9.3 g, Fiber: 7.2 g

Chocolate And Walnut Farfalle

Preparation time: 10 minutes

cooking time: 0 minutes

servings: 4

Ingredients

- 8 ounces farfalle
- 1/2 cup chopped toasted walnuts
- 1/4 cup vegan semisweet chocolate pieces
- 3 tablespoons vegan margarine
- 1/4 cup light brown sugar

Directions

1. In a food processor or blender, grind the walnuts and chocolate pieces until crumbly. Do not overprocess. Set aside.
2. In a pot of boiling salted water, cook the farfalle, stirring occasionally, until al dente, about 8 minutes. Drain well and return to the pot.
3. Add the margarine and sugar and toss to combine and melt the margarine.
4. Transfer the noodle mixture to a serving

Almond-Date Energy Bites

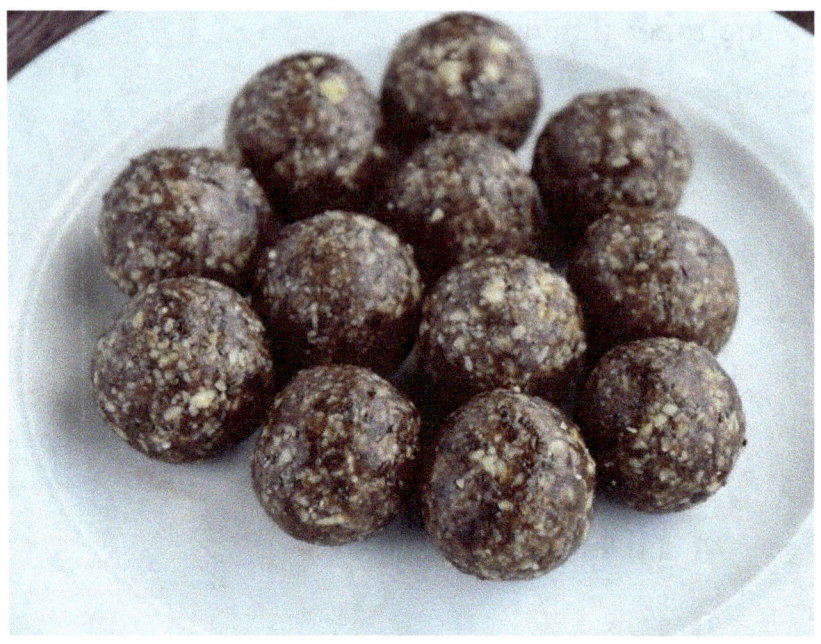

Preparation time: 5 minutes • chill time: 15 minutes servings: 24 bites

Ingredients

- ¼ cup chia seeds
- 1 cup dates, pitted
- 1 cup unsweetened shredded coconut
- ¾ cup ground almonds
- ¼ cup cocoa nibs, or non-dairy chocolate chips

Directions

1. Purée everything in a food processor until crumbly and sticking together, pushing down the sides whenever necessary to keep it blending. If you don't have a food processor, you can mash soft Medjool dates. But if you're using harder baking dates, you'll have to soak them and then try to purée them in a blender.
2. Form the mix into 24 balls and place them on a baking sheet lined with parchment or waxed paper. Put in the fridge to set for about 15 minutes. Use the softest dates you can find. Medjool dates are the best for this purpose. The hard dates you see in the baking aisle of your supermarket are going to take a long time to blend up. If you use those, try soaking them in water for at least an hour before you start, and then draining.

Nutrition (1 bite)

Calories: 152; Total fat: 11g; Carbs: 13g; Fiber: 5g; Protein: 3g

Melon Coconut Mousse

Preparation time: 10 minutes

Cooking time: 0 minutes

Servings: 6

Ingredients:

- 2 cups coconut cream
- 1 teaspoon vanilla extract
- 1 tablespoon stevia
- 1 cup melon, peeled and chopped

Directions:

1. In a blender, combine the melon with the cream and the other ingredients, pulse well, divide into bowls and serve cold.

Nutrition:

Calories 219, fat 21.1, fiber 0.9, carbs 7, protein 1.4

Chia Seeds Pudding with Berries

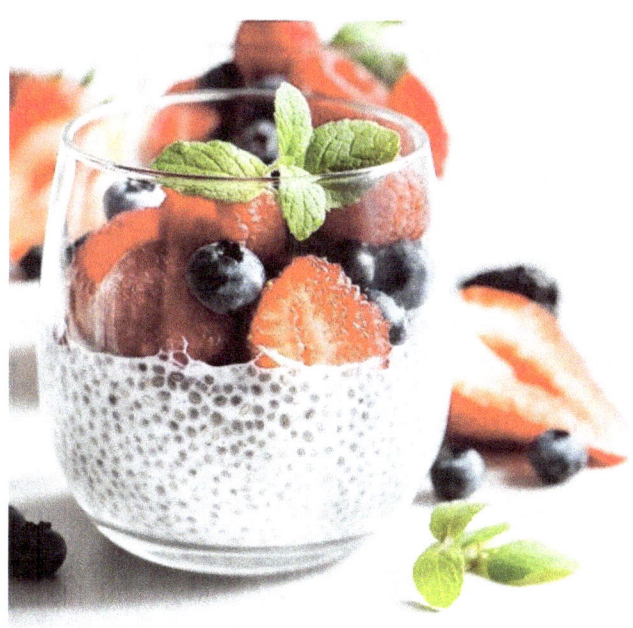

Preparation time: 60 minutes

Ingredients:

- ½ cups chia seeds
- 2 cups coconut milk, full fat
- 1 banana, sliced
- Honey or stevia for sweetening
- 5 Oz. at least any fresh berries

Directions:

1. Stir the milk, chia seeds and stevia (or honey) in a mixing bowl.
2. Add half of all the berries and let the mixture chilled for at least 1 hour.
3. Mix it up again and add the berries and banana before serving.

Tip: Chia seeds have omega-3 fatty acids, protein, fiber, calcium and antioxidants.

Dates and Cocoa Bowls

Preparation time: 2 hours

Cooking time: 0 minutes

Servings: 6

Ingredients:

- 1 teaspoon cocoa powder
- 2 tablespoons avocado oil
- 1 cup coconut cream
- ½ cup dates, chopped
- 3 tablespoons stevia

Directions:

1. In a bowl, mix the cream with the oil, the cocoa, the cream and the other ingredients, pulse well, divide into cups and keep in the fridge for 2 hours before serving.

Nutrition:

Calories 141, fat 10.2, fiber 2.4, carbs 13.8, protein 1.4

Blackberries Brownies

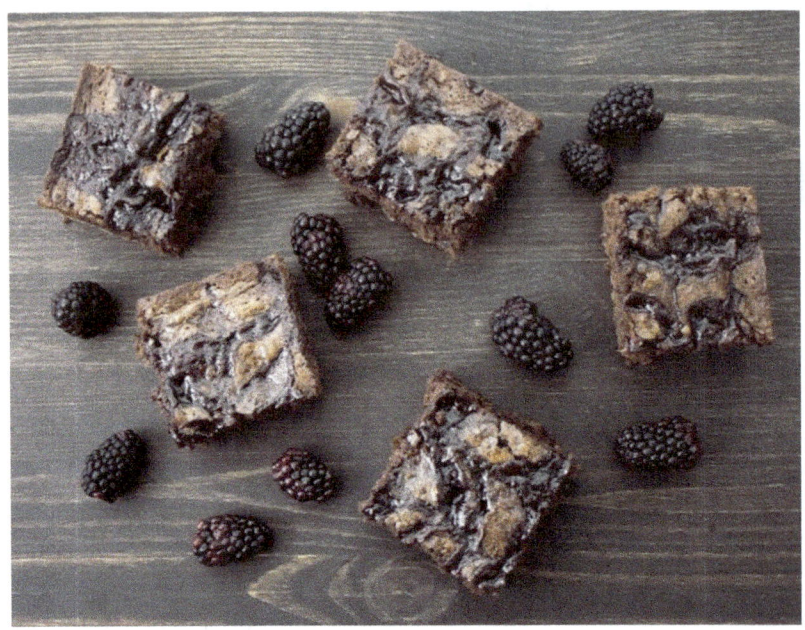

Preparation time: 10 minutes

Cooking time: 20 minutes

Servings: 8

Ingredients:

- 1 cup almond flour
- 1 cup blackberries
- 1 avocado, peeled, pitted and chopped
- ½ teaspoon baking soda

- 4 tablespoons coconut oil, melted
- 1 tablespoon stevia
- 2 tablespoons lime zest, grated
- Cooking spray

Directions:

1. In a food processor, combine the flour with the blackberries and the other ingredients except the cooking spray and pulse well.
2. Pour this into a pan greased with cooking spray, spread evenly, introduce in the oven at 380 degrees F and bake for 20 minutes.
3. Cut the brownies and serve cold.

Nutrition:

Calories 200, fat 4.5, fiber 2.4 carbs 8.7, protein 4.3

Rhubarb Stew

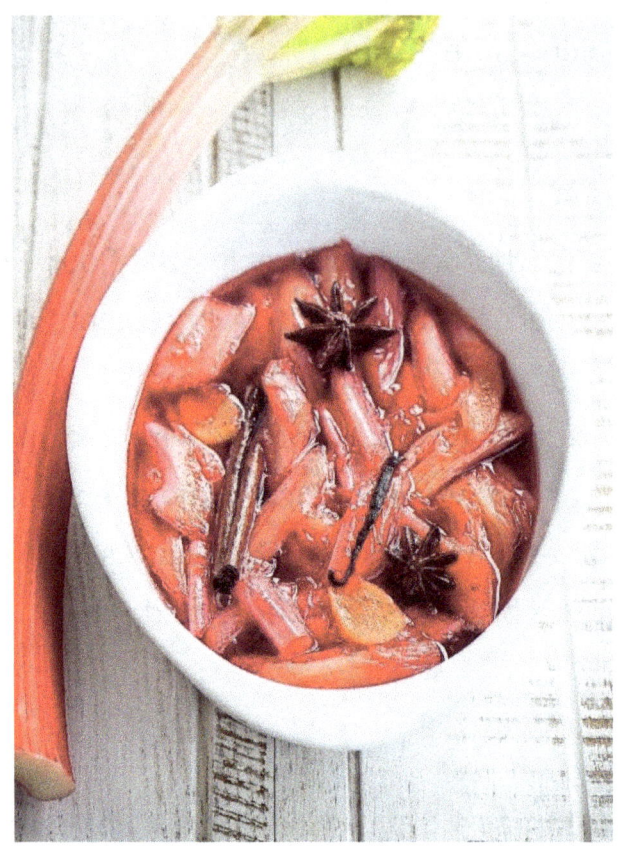

Preparation time: 10 minutes

Cooking time: 10 minutes

Servings: 4

Ingredients:

- 2 tablespoons stevia
- Juice of ½ lemon
- 1 cup water
- 1 teaspoon vanilla extract
- 1 teaspoon lemon zest, grated
- 2 cups rhubarb, roughly chopped

Directions:

1. Heat up a pan with the water over medium heat, add the stevia, the rhubarb and the other ingredients, toss, simmer for 10 minutes, divide into cups and serve cold.

Nutrition:

Calories 122, fat 3.7, fiber 1.2, carbs 2.3, protein 0.4

Cocoa Cream

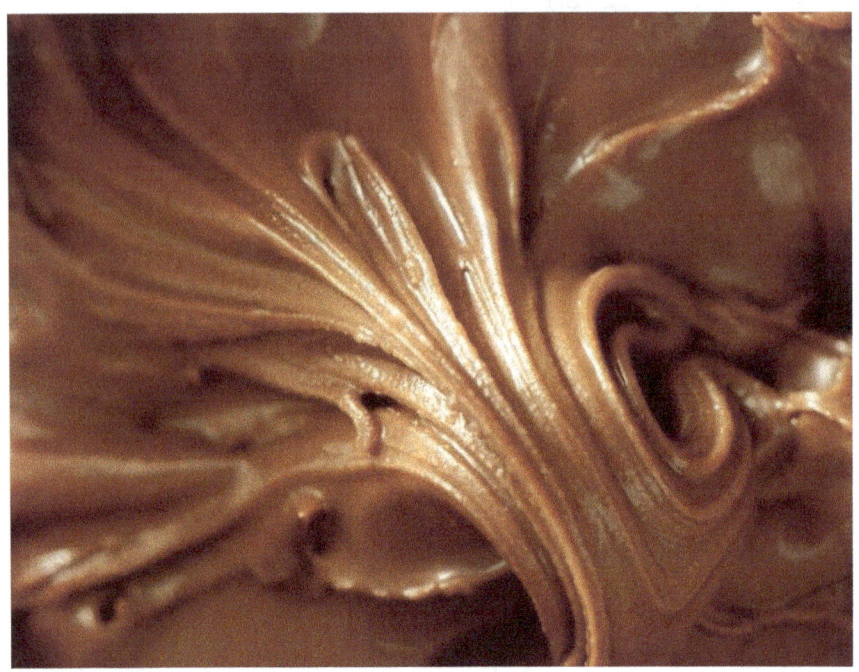

Preparation time: 2 hours

Cooking time: 0 minutes

Servings: 4

Ingredients:

- ½ cup cocoa powder
- ¾ cup coconut cream

- 1 teaspoon cinnamon powder
- ¼ cup stevia
- 1 teaspoon vanilla extract

Directions:

1. In a blender, mix the cream with the cocoa powder, stevia and the other ingredients, pulse well, divide into cups and keep in the fridge for 2 hours before serving.

Nutrition:

Calories 162, fat 3.4, fiber 2.4, carbs 5, protein 1

Cloud Bread

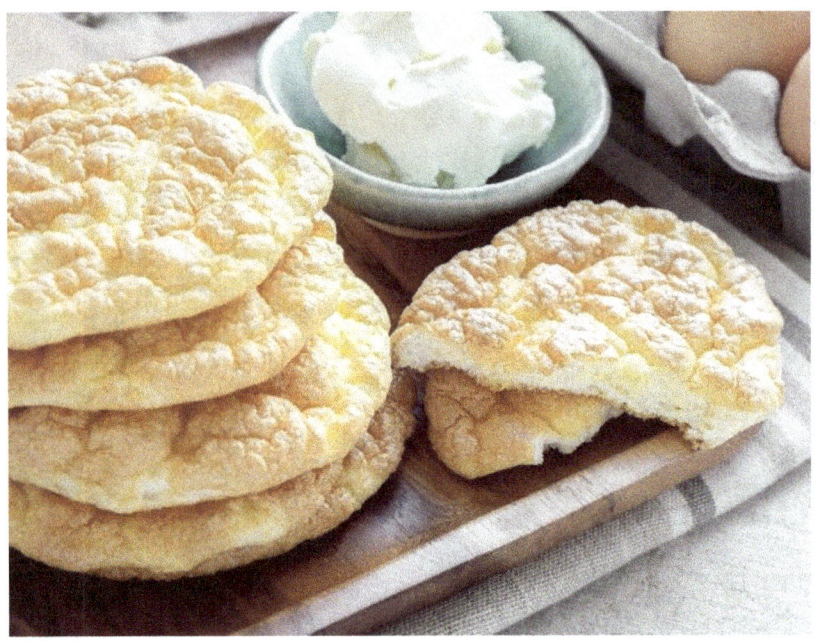

Preparation time: 15 minutes

Cooking time: 35 minutes

Servings: 6

Ingredients:

- Nonstick cooking spray
- 3 eggs, separated, at room temperature
- 3 ounces cream cheese, at room temperature

- ⅛ teaspoon salt

Directions:

1. Preheat the oven to 300 °F. Spray a baking sheet with cooking spray.
2. In a large mixing bowl, use a handheld electric mixer to beat the egg whites into stiff peaks. Set aside.
3. In a separate large bowl, combine the egg yolks, cream cheese, and salt, and mix until creamy.
4. Slowly pour the egg white mixture into the egg yolk mixture, and use a spatula to fold it in carefully. Be careful not to overmix.
5. Use the batter to make 6 separate circles on the prepared baking sheet. These will be your clouds.
6. Bake for 30 to 35 minutes or until golden brown.
7. Remove from the oven and allow to cool for 10 minutes before serving.

nutrition:

Calories 82, fat 7g, protein 4g, carbs 1g, fiber 0g, sugar 0g, sodium 123mg

Simple Almond Butter Fudge

Preparation Time: 15 minutes

Cooking Time: 0 minute

Servings: 8

Ingredients:

- 1/2 cup almond butter
- 15 drops liquid stevia
- 2 1/2 tbsp coconut oil

Directions:

1. Combine together almond butter and coconut oil in a saucepan. Gently warm until melted.
2. Add stevia and stir well.
3. Pour mixture into the candy container and place in refrigerator until set.
4. Serve and enjoy.

nutrition:

Calories 43, Fat 4.8g, Carbohydrates 0.2g, Protein 0.2g, Sugars 0g, Cholesterol 0mg

Choco Chia Pudding

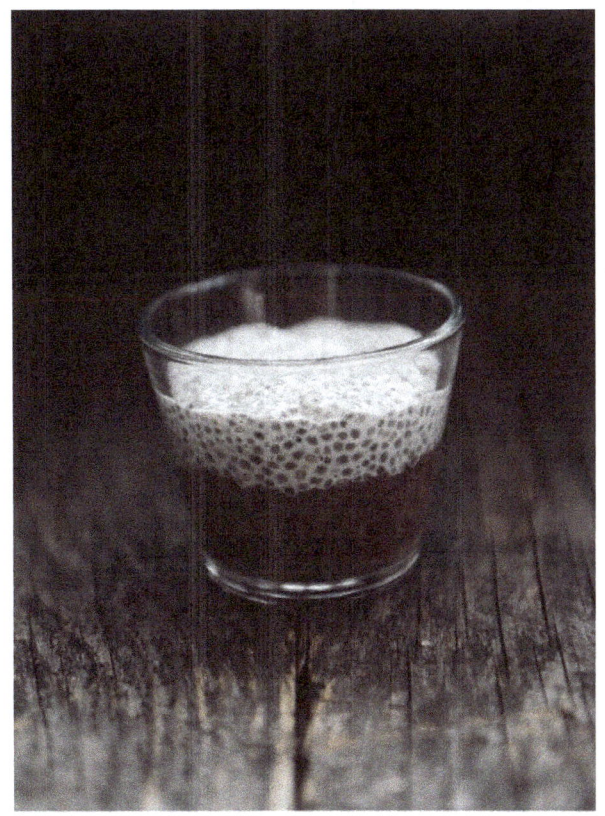

Preparation Time: 10 minutes

Cooking Time: 0 minute

Servings: 6

Ingredients:

- 2 1/2 cups coconut milk
- 1/2 cup chia seeds
- 2 scoops stevia extract powder
- 6 tbsp cocoa powder
- 1/2 tsp vanilla extract
- 1/8 cup xylitol
- 1/8 tsp salt

Directions:

1. Add all ingredients into the blender and blend until smooth.
2. Pour mixture into the glass container and place in the refrigerator.
3. Serve chilled and enjoy.

nutrition:

Calories 259, Fat 25.4g, Carbohydrates 10.2g, Sugar 3.5g, Protein 3.8g, Cholesterol 0mg

NOTE

www.ingramcontent.com/pod-product-compliance
Lightning Source LLC
Chambersburg PA
CBHW072205100526
44589CB00015B/2381